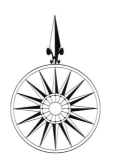

North *of* Shadowlands

LETTERS FROM A SERIOUS ILLNESS
DERICK BINGHAM

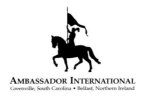

AMBASSADOR INTERNATIONAL
Greenville, South Carolina • Belfast, Northern Ireland

North of Shadowlands
LETTERS FROM A SERIOUS ILLNESS

© Copyright 2009 Derick Bingham

Scripture taken from the Holy Bible, New international Version® NIV.
Copyright ©1973,1978,1984 by International Bible Society.
Used by permission of Zondervan Publishing House. All rights reserved.

ISBN 978-1-84030-219-6

Ambassador Publications
a division of
Ambassador Productions Ltd.
Providence House
Ardenlee Street,
Belfast,
BT6 8QJ
Northern Ireland
www.ambassador-productions.com

Emerald House
427 Wade Hampton Blvd.
Greenville
SC 29609, USA
www.emeraldhouse.com

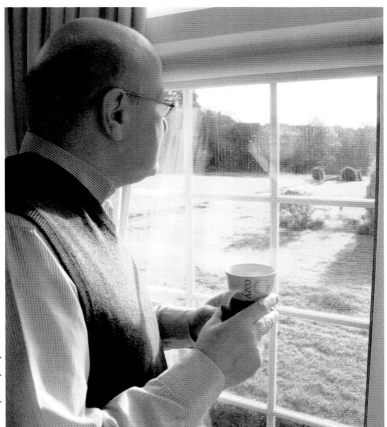

*- This book of letters is dedicated to
Hampton and Sharon Hewitt
whose kindness to us is
beyond articulating -*

Many thanks to Dorothy Boyd for collating the letters
for this book and to my friends at ChristChurch
who originally posted them on the Net.

'Don't lose the letters', he said. Who is he? He is a friend of mine who is, believe me, not given to sentiment. As one of the founders of the Irish Association of Dermatologists, Professor Desmond Burrows has a long and distinguished career in medicine behind him. This summer, it gave the people of Northern Ireland - and others across the world - great pleasure to learn that he had been awarded the Sir Archibald Gray Gold Medal. This is the highest accolade of the British Association of Dermatologists, and is awarded for an outstanding contribution to British Dermatology.

He had obviously been reading my letters on our church blog. This blog was kindly set up for me by our church to inform people who had been enquiring about my condition after I had been diagnosed with Acute Myeloid Leukaemia (Leukemia in the United States).

My friend was very keen that I publish my blog letters. I put up an argument against it and he immediately demolished it, arguing that he was convinced the letters would help people who were seriously ill. From such a person I knew the plea was not idle conversation. This book is honouring that plea.

These letters were written in the raw across extremely distressing days and nights and therefore I have added some footnotes to fill in necessary, and I hope, helpful details. What the letters lack in literary value, I hope they will make up for in directness of heart-to-heart communication. If my letters become as a signpost pointing anyone to go for help to the Conqueror of Death, I will be overjoyed.

In the fellowship of the easy yoke,

Derick Bingham

Belfast, Christmas 2009

'Never knew so long a spell of fogs. One pines for lights and, scarcely less, shadows, which make up so much of the beauty of the world'

C.S. Lewis

Letters to an American Lady

(Hodder and Stoughton 1967)

Saturday 7th MARCH, 2009

Dear everyone,

Two weeks ago, while serving the Lord at the Tobermore Bible Week,[1] I began to feel extremely unwell. After taking two Sunday morning services, I found my appetite slipping, and at the home of the Rev John Flaherty, the gifted Presbyterian minister of Draperstown and Tobermore Presbyterian Churches, I excused myself from the dinner table and asked if I could sleep. I fell into a very deep sleep and, somewhat refreshed, rose to take the evening service. By suppertime I felt very unwell.

I made it home with Margaret to Belfast, and the next morning, noticing my extreme weakness, she called in the Doctor. He immediately admitted me by ambulance to the Belfast City Hospital, where I was shortly diagnosed with Acute Myeloid Leukaemia. The medical Professor in charge of my case gently made it clear to me that I had but a few days to live.

The Professor offered me chemotherapy, but left the choice entirely with me as to whether to take it or not.[2]

In my extreme weakness - and it was a very dark place - I wondered if I should slip away to be with Christ, who's face I long to see. Thinking of you all and above everything else my beloved family, and with the godly council of the

---

1. Held each year by the combined congregations of the Baptist, Presbyterian, and Church of Ireland congregations in Tobermore, County Londonderry.
2. Later she informed me there had been a deep discussion between the six doctors looking after me. Three wanted to give me the Chemo; three others didn't because they thought my body would not take it. The decision was left to me.

hospital Chaplain, the Rev Muriel Cromie,[3] who has long attended my ministry across many years, I decided, in the words of Robert Browning the poet, to go for 'one fight more, the best and the last'[4].

I have found death stalking me for days, and he is certainly no friend but an enemy. Strangely, through the darkest first few nights, I found myself singing beautiful hymns to my beautiful Saviour, the Conqueror of Death. Being a writer who is a committed Christian, I kept thinking of the dying Romantic poet John Keats. He had a friend called Joseph Severn who cared for him in his dying hours. One day he said to him 'I can't believe in your book, the Bible. But I feel a horrible want of some faith-some hope-something to rest on now?'[5]

Severn went, at Keats's request, and got him a copy of the *Pilgrim's Progress* by John Bunyan and Jeremy Taylor's *Holy Living and Holy Dying*.[6] Severn always believed Keats came to faith before he died.

I have not the slightest doubt whatsoever that the Scriptures are the unbreakable, inerrant word of the living God, and the comfort they have brought me in this howling storm is beyond human reason.

Day after day messages pour in from people from the most varied walks of life. It has been an overwhelming experience. Across my life I have sought to teach God's word, and I am now discovering through the messages sent to me that an incredible harvest has been brought about by the seeds sown.

3. Rev. Muriel Cromie, Presbyterian Chaplain to the Belfast City Hospital. She told me that I owed it to my family and all who I had ministered to across the years to stay awhile longer (she called it 'your legacy, Derick!!'). She did not tell me to take the Chemo but I got her drift. She was as an Angel from Heaven to me. My son-in-law, David, also wonderfully inspired me by holding up Lance Armstrong of Tour de France fame who has so bravely fought cancer seven times!

4. Robert Browning, Prospice, 1861. One of my favourite poems on the subject of death.

5. Joseph Severn to John Taylor, Rome 24th Dec.1820. Source: english history.net/keats/letters/severn2.html I was deeply aware that in Christ I had something to rest on.

6. Jeremy Taylor was appointed Bishop of Down and Connor in Ireland by Charles II and built Dromore Cathedral in Co. Down.

A man even sent his young son who is a Doctor in this hospital to tell me he had found Christ when he was a student at Queen's University at 'Tuesday Night at the Crescent'[7]. The lady who washes me had attended the same meetings. The lady in charge of my CT scan happily told me of the days she used to go too. On and on it goes. As the book of Ruth puts it, my heavenly Boaz has dropped me 'handfuls of purpose'[8] day after day in this dark, dark place of suffering.

Thank you to all of you who have inquired after me and shown kindnesses to my family. Because of the extreme risk of infection, it is highly dangerous for me to have visitors. Just keep praying for me. Thank you all for your love. I have discovered that I am more loved than I ever imagined, and I am deeply humbled by it.

The medical team tells me my first course of chemotherapy has done exactly what they expected to date. My white cell count is now normal. They have warned me that there are still very rough days ahead. Can I just say that I have not the slightest iota of bitterness towards God? I have been deeply inspired by the famous line written by Amy Carmichael, my beloved hero: 'In acceptance lieth peace'[9]. I humbly and by faith accept God's good and perfect will.

In the fellowship of the easy yoke,
Derick Bingham

---

7. A weekly Bible Class I had the privilege of teaching for 21 years at the Crescent Church in the University District of South Belfast.

8. Ruth 2:16 Authorized Version

9. See my biography of Amy Carmichael, 'The Wild-Bird Child', Ambassador International. She was an invalid in the same room for 23 years.

'Faith means believing in advance what only makes sense in reverse'

Philip Yancey
Disappointment with God
(Zondervan 1997)

Sunday 15th MARCH, 2009
THE SUN COMING UP IN THE MORNING

Dear everyone,

Warm Greetings. I am now approaching the end of my third week in Ward 10 in the Belfast City Hospital, following my diagnosis of Acute Myeloid Leukaemia, which fell on me like a meteor out of the sky. The care and attention given me by the medical team here is incredibly skilled, always dedicated and, for me, deeply humbling to receive. This place has the reputation of being one of the greatest cancer centre's in Europe - and I believe it.

Often, not having the strength to lift hand or foot, especially when my hemoglobin is low, I am watched and ministered to at all times.

My first course of Chemo is over, and I am now waiting to see if the 'good' cells will grow back, now that the cancerous cells have been successfully driven back. I am massively open to infection.

Almost daily I have been inspired by the visits of Professor Jim Dornan,[10] a longstanding friend of mine, who also delivered all of my children and my grandson at birth. He has Leukaemia and has successfully fought it. He comes to see me early in the morning before he goes to his famous maternity clinic at the Royal Victoria Hospital. To be quite honest, he is like the sun coming up every morning!

10. Director of Fetal Medicine at the Royal Maternity Hospital, Belfast and was Senior Vice-President International of the Royal College of Obstetricians and Gynecologists. He got down on his knees by my bedside in the isolation ward, took me by the arm and said 'You've got to fight it, Derick!' Those words were gold dust to me as I began to understand that the darker mental side of my disease needed to be mentally fought.

I had no idea how Chemo can affect one mentally, and Jim drives me on to fight the dark mental side of this disease. Despite his condition, he recently sailed a yacht across the Atlantic, along with a few friends. Having such a person by one's bed every morning cannot but give you the 'Audacity of Hope', as President Obama would put it. He has also prayed fervently with me and for me.

I have also appreciated deeply the kind and helpful ministry of the two Hospital Chaplains, the Rev. Muriel Cromie and Mr. Edward Jamison.[11]

Another thing that has surprised me greatly has been the discovery that I am loved at a very deep level both by a great number of people at home in Northern Ireland and over the hills and far away. Through the kindness of my church family, a website has been opened for people to send a message to me. I am overwhelmed by the expressions of love for me that have been poured out. Christian ministry is often a very lonely work indeed, and one is not always aware of the effect it is having, or has had, in the hand of God. Now through these comments the Lord has graciously revealed to me that His Word which I have been privileged to preach and teach has borne a harvest above all I could have undeservedly asked or thought. I first started preaching God's Word when I was a lad of twelve,[12] and have been doing it most weekends ever since. I am now 62.

The letters and cards that have poured in, mentioning passages of Scripture I have been privileged to teach or write about in my books, and how these have touched lives, is a glorious sight for my weary eyes. I mention this to encourage all of you who teach and communicate the Scriptures. Your work is anything but insignificant, and has eternal repercussions.

---

11. Former Christian missionary to Bolivia.
12. It all began when I was asked to give my Christian testimony in services. I usually wore my Down High School uniform!

I have always loved the testimony of J.B. Phillips, when he set out to write a modern translation of the Scriptures. He said 'it was like trying to rewire an ancient house without being able to switch off the mains.'[12] Thank you to all of you who have unashamedly expressed your love for me. You have heartened one of my darkest hours.

I am writing this through the wee hours of the morning. I cannot sleep much tonight, and would like to point out some things before I try to sleep again.

I have been thinking much over these very difficult and uncertain days about the humanist advertisement on buses which points out that, from their point of view, it is reasonable to believe that there is no God. They advise that we go and enjoy ourselves. Now if this were true, where would I go? I am not permitted to go anywhere outside this hospital room and ward at the present time. Where then can I find enjoyment? I find it in the Lord Jesus. He has given me real 'Bread from Heaven.' He restores my soul. He is a hidden source of deep, refreshing Living Water from which I draw. As Samuel Rutherford said 'Christ is lovely, He is always lovely, He is altogether lovely.' At his right hand are pleasures forever more.[14]

It is often very difficult to concentrate to read and pray in my present condition - though as you can see, this is improving gradually for me. The very first passage of Scripture I was able to read since coming here was 1 Peter 1, which suddenly rose powerfully in my mind. It tells me what I have as a Christian. It was, of course, written by a man who, like me, often failed to live up to his high Christian profession.

13. 'Translating the Gospels: A Discussion between Dr E.V. Rieu and Rev J.B. Phillips', The Bible Translator (Oct 1955).
14. Psalm 16:11

From a resurrected Saviour, who made him breakfast by a lake one morning, Peter discovered that neither failure, nor mood nor time would ever change his Master's love and commitment to him. By the way, it is worth remembering with regard to Christ's resurrection, that the greatest news the world ever heard came from a graveyard![15]

'Praise be to the God and Father of our Lord Jesus Christ! In His great mercy,' writes Peter, 'He has given us new birth into a living hope through the resurrection of Jesus Christ from the dead'. So as a Christian I have a living hope. How many of my hopes have I had to bury? Many. This one, though, I will never have to bury because it is living.

And, writes Peter, 'into an inheritance that can never perish, spoil or fade reserved in heaven for you'. As a Christian I have an incorruptible inheritance. As the world economy collapses, as millions lose employment, as wealth flies away like an eagle in a storm, none of this can touch my inheritance in Christ.[16]

Even as death stalked me in my first Chemo course - it was touch and go but I made it, I was told I had a five percent chance of surviving - through it all my inheritance reserved for me was untouchable by anything.

'Who through faith are shielded by God's power until the coming of the salvation that is ready to be revealed in the last time', says Peter. So I am also shielded by God's power, which is the best shield a fellow could possibly have.

And my present condition? 'In this you greatly rejoice', writes Peter, 'though now for a little while you have had to suffer grief in all kinds of trials. These have come so that your faith - of greater worth than gold, which perishes even though refined by fire - may prove to be genuine and may result in praise, glory and honour when Jesus Christ is revealed. Though you have not seen

---

15. Matthew 28:1-7

16. The financial crises of 2007-2009 has been called by leading economists the worst financial crisis since the one related to the Great Depression in the decade preceding World War 11.

him you love him and even though you do not see him now, you believe in him and are filled with an inexpressible and glorious joy for you are receiving the goal of your faith, the salvation of your souls'.

How can one best sum up this complex situation? This week my daughter passed on to me this wonderful quote from Philip Yancey. 'Faith is believing in advance what only makes sense in reverse'.

Onward!
Derick Bingham

The Dawning

Awake, sad heart, which sorrow ever drowns;
Take up thine eyes, which feed on earth;
Unfold thy forehead gathered into frowns:
Thy Saviour comes, and with Him mirth:
Awake, awake,
And with a thankful heart his comforts take.
But thou dost still lament, and pine, and cry,
And feel his death, but not his victory.

Arise sad heart; if thou dost not withstand,
Christ's resurrection thine may be;
Do not by hanging down break from the hand,
Which, as it riseth, raiseth thee:
Arise, Arise;
And with his burial linen dry thine eyes.
Christ left his grave-clothes, that we might, when grief
Draws tears, or blood, not want an handkerchief.

From *The Temple* collection of poems
by George Herbert (1593-1633).

George Herbert was appointed Reader in Rhetoric at Cambridge in 1618, and in 1620 was elected to the post of Cambridge University orator, holding this position until 1628. He served as a Member of Parliament for two years (1624-1626) and entered the Anglican ministry in 1630 serving as a rector of the little parish of St Andrew Bemerton, near Salisbury, in Wiltshire. He suffered from poor health and died from tuberculosis three years later. He reportedly gave the manuscript of The Temple to a friend on his deathbed, telling him to publish the poems if he thought they might 'turn to the advantage of any dejected soul', and otherwise, to burn them. I discovered a quotation of the last two lines of this beautiful poem while in hospital at Easter 2009 (376 years later!). They meant more to me than I can express.

That Easter morning my friend Edward Fitzgerald and I were the only two patients on the hospital ward. We held an Easter service together rejoicing in the fact that Christ said that where two or three were gathered in his name he would be 'in the midst'. I read the Easter story from the Scriptures and Edward prayed. It was one of the best Easter services I have ever been in!!

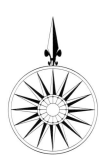

Wednesday 8th APRIL, 2009
EASTER LETTER

Dear everyone,

Warm Greetings.

Spring sunshine, Margaret's incredibly, unbelievably delicious cooking, a walk by Hillsborough Lake, the smell of spring flowers, the inexpressible sight of my grandchildren Jamie and Sophie playing Lego around my feet, time to sit and talk at ease with my incredibly loving family; I feel like following Kenneth Grahame's 'Moley' who headed out of Mole End one fine Spring day where 'it all seemed too good to be true. Hither and thither through the meadows, he rambled busily, along the hedgerows, across the copses, finding everywhere birds building, flowers budding, leaves thrusting - everything happy, progressive and occupied.'[17]

I cannot really describe how wonderful it is to be home for an extended period, free from Chemo, catheters, blood transfusions, platelet transfusions, morphine etc (all so skilfully given) and long, long, seemingly interminable nights. I almost feel like saying to my grandchildren with Helen Oxenbury and Michael Rosin: 'We're going on a bear hunt/ We're are going to catch a big one/ What a beautiful day!'[18] Whatever the future holds for me, it truly is blissful to be home, and I am relishing every moment of it.

I am now waiting for a call to go back into hospital for my next Chemo course, probably beginning next week. In the meantime I am euphoric at being

17. Kenneth Graham, 'The Wind in the Willows', originally published by Metheun & Co Ltd, 1908.
18. Michael Rosin and Helen Oxbury, 'We're Going on a Bear Hunt', Walker Books Ltd, 1997.

home. My friend Canon David Jardine, who has ministered to my spiritual needs across many days, calls it 'a miracle'.[19] The medical team caring for me call it 'remission', but I humbly call it 'permission', and may I glorify the Lord in every way I can in whatever days he has spared me to live. The winds were contrary to me, but they were not contrary to the Lord, as he walked into another storm and pulled another child of his out of the water, as I desperately sought to meet him in the darkness. Not forgetting, of course, that Peter, when it happened to him, had more storms to face. But, my, how Peter later had the victory in those storms because of that experience in the Galilee storm.

Just recently I received a card from my godly and much loved colleague Dr. Hadden Wilson, gently hoping I would share what God is teaching me (changing the metaphor) 'in the furnace' of my present experience. Dr. Wilson is Pastor Emeritus of Ballynahinch Baptist Church and Honorary Studies Co-ordinator in Ireland for John Brown University. One thing is for sure, like Daniel's three friends, in this furnace I have experienced the presence of another 'like unto the Son of God.' I have no idea where this experience of Acute Myeloid Leukaemia is heading, but I do know that my awesome Lord and Saviour is coming with me.

I have been musing on the moving story of those bewildered, disillusioned, sad, lonely disciples, heading home to their village home in Emmaus, after the momentous events surrounding Christ's death at Jerusalem. Perhaps the best word to describe their condition was that they were confused about their circumstances - where was this one they had implicitly trusted? Where were his promises, mind-boggling in their implications

19. David along with others founded Divine Healing Ministries in 1992 which has since then, on an interdenominational basis, prayed for the healing of individuals and our land. David who was at Down High School with me, brought me deep comfort and encouragement and with godly earnestness, anointed me with oil in hospital.

for the future of mankind, the earth and the universe? Then the resurrected maker of galaxies and little children, the one who protects precious seed covered in the snows of winter, and resurrects it in the exploding, indescribable cascading beauty of spring, joined those two saddened disciples on that road with all of their questions. Here was no bombastic, self-seeking earthly celebrity, famous for simply being famous. Here, rather, was the Light from behind the sun, resurrected from the dead. As has been said, 'the stone was not rolled away from the tomb of the Lord Jesus to let him out, it was rolled away to let his followers in!'[20]

How like him, though, not to throw his awesome power around in some earth shattering action, but to come gently alongside his confused disciples to eradicate their fear and doubts in such a human way. He asked them what they had been discussing together as they had been walking along. I have been thinking on how we are told that the two men stood still, their faces downcast. 'Are you only a visitor to Jerusalem and do not know the things that have happened there in these days?' they said. 'What things?' asked the one at whose word the Universe was created; he who spoke to nothing and it became something so complex and incredible in the face of which even the greatest of human minds can only stagger. As the men stood still (not knowing who stood beside them) they began to pour out all their hearts and honest disillusionment. I am sure they thought it was the worst day of their lives. Actually, though they did not yet know it, it would turn out to be their best.

Then came the 'visitor's' unequivocal reprimand, speaking right to the heart of their faltering faith: 'How foolish you are, and how slow of heart to believe all that the prophets have spoken! Did not Christ have to suffer these things and then enter his glory? And beginning at Moses and all the prophets, he explained to them what was said in all the Scriptures concerning himself.'

---

20. Matthew 28:2

Could I digress for a wee minute? The other day I listened to Kirsty Young interview Sebastian Faulk, the great novelist (*Birdsong* etc) on Radio 4's Desert Island Discs. He spoke of his life as a writer, of whiskey and jazz and family, his love of history, and the things that really mattered to him. He then spoke of the death of his father whom he greatly respected, and of a Requiem that had had been sung at his father's funeral. He chose the Requiem for one of his Desert Island discs (Requiem, Op 48 iii Sanctus, sung by the choir of St John's College, Cambridge) and then made the amazing and moving statement that there were those who had faith to believe that everything would turn out well in a redemptive end. He said he did not have such a faith, but envied those who did. The atheist writer Thomas Hardy said exactly the same thing in his haunting poem *The Funeral of God.*

Oh Sebastian, Britain, and particularly Western Europe as a whole 'How foolish you are, and how slow of heart to believe all that the prophets have spoken' of Christ, his redemptive sacrifice and freely offered forgiveness and salvation to all who repent toward God and have faith in him. It could be yours, millions of you! Just look at China with its 30 million plus believers and the vast swathes of Africa where millions have turned to Christ for the good. If you doubt me, just go and read Mathew Parris's article *As an atheist I truly believe Africa needs God* (*The Times* online, published 27th December 2008).

To return to our story, we are told that as the end of the day came after their seven-mile walk, the disciples invited the Lord Jesus into their home in Emmaus to stay with them. It turned out to be one of the most poignant moments in history, when, as the Saviour of the world thanked God for the bread on the supper table, the disciple's eyes were opened and they recognised him. He disappeared, but now the two men spoke of how their hearts had burned within them while the Lord opened the Scriptures to them as they had talked on the road. They headed back up to Jerusalem that very evening filled with joy. They walked along the very same road, but were very different men from the ones who had come down it.

As I have lain on my back for about 36 days in hospital, I have, of course, been reviewing my life, my sad failures and faults and sins, and, of course, the wonderful forgiveness and victories I have had in Christ. As I have lain there, I have been thinking of the places across the world where I have been undeservedly privileged to teach God's Word for three decades and more, and of the great things the Lord has done. From Ballywillwill to Bucharest, from Oxford to Osaka, from Lerwick to Keswick, from Rosemary Lane to Ronnie Heron's barn, from Cuthbert, Georgia to the Crescent Church through hundreds of Tuesday nights, from Bible classes in Newtownards, Glasgow and Edinburgh and many, many weekends in Ayr, in homes, in children's missions, in universities, in schools, in the open air, in the Royal Albert Hall and Capernwray Hall (Oh for a coffee in the Beehive!), from the last ten years with ChristChurch, Belfast to nine weeks in Korea with Margaret as I sought to reach out with the Word of God to many Korean people by radio broadcasts and in a stadium in the heart of Seoul. In all kinds of diverse corners of the world, and situations as varied as the people in them, I have found something in common with them all. As I have taught God's inerrant word, a moment always comes of silent awesome recognition (even with children), that when the Bible speaks, God is speaking. Recognition comes that it is no longer just the preacher's voice to which they are listening, but God's voice. In fact, Billy Graham has said that the preacher is not really preaching until the listener hears another voice.

It is for many the very same thing as those two men experienced on the Emmaus road, when they heard Christ explain what was said in all the

Scriptures concerning himself: their hearts burned. As John Wesley most famously put it, when he listened to Romans being expounded on the night of his conversion: his heart was 'strangely warmed.'[21] Ah! When self is forgotten, and the Spirit of God fills the Bible communicator by coffee table or public pulpit or wherever, there is nothing on earth more effective to the transformation of lives and the glorification of Christ and his kingdom. I know that preaching and teaching and communicating God's Word is, at this time in the Western word, often at low ebb… but may it return soon in power. As CH Spurgeon said 'you don't need to defend a lion – just let him loose!!'

I was once kindly loaned a model of the Tabernacle by my friend Professor David Gooding,[22] and I spent many hours teaching across those forty chapters given to the Tabernacle in the Old Testament at my Bible classes at the Crescent Church as well as in 'Greek Thompson's' famous and beautiful church building on St Vincent Street Glasgow. Professor Gooding quietly said to me one day 'When you teach this you will find Heaven will descend.' He never spoke more truthful words. If you doubt me in this year of anniversary of the great 1859 Revival in Ireland, just ask the present Minster of Connor Presbyterian Church in Kells, Co. Antrim. His church building was built to accommodate the converts at that time, and he will tell you of an unforgettable

---

21. 'In the evening I went very unwillingly to a society in Aldersgate Street, where one was reading Luther's preface to the Epistle to the Romans. About a quarter before nine he was describing the change which God works in the heart through faith in Christ. I felt my heart strangely warmed. I felt I did trust in Christ, Christ alone, for salvation; and an assurance was given me, that he had taken away my sins, even mine, and saved me from the law of sin and death' (John Wesley/ from his personal Journal which he kept from October 1735 to October 1790).

22. International author and Professor Emeritus of O.T.Greek at Queen's University of Belfast and a member of the Royal Irish Academy. Across my life David has selflessly given me many, many hours of his time to privately open up the Scriptures to me. I could never repay the debt I owe him. I shall never forget the day in his home when in one of his private teaching sessions I had to ask him to stop as I wanted to bow my head and worship God. He had shown me God as revealed in his Word and I worshipped. With all my heart I recommend his books to anyone.

night when, far from God, he came to hear teaching at 'Tuesday Night at the Crescent' on the Tabernacle, and was incredibly converted on the very first night he came (bless him and his ministry!)

How, of course, could I ever have been able to see all this without my wife Margaret? The years she has given of holding down our home so incredibly smoothly, through unending pressure, only the Lord truly knows about. Her dedication was and is absolute, and she has been a luxury to love. My longsuffering and loving children, Kathryn, Kerrie and Claire deserve a reward greater than I could ever give them - but the Lord will give it to them.

So, then, rising generation of Christians, back to the Word. Trust it, believe it, live it, preach it, teach and communicate it, and Europe can once more know days of huge revival in the church, and spiritual awakening in the nations. Not forgetting, of course, that the Word leads to the living Word our Lord Jesus himself.

As for me, I am heading down my Emmaus road, not knowing if my Lord will now lead me to glory, or back to more service for him in preaching and teaching his Word. I simply do not know what is going to happen. But I do know one thing, put perfectly by the Rev. Murray McCheyne: We are immortal until our work is done. As the American writer Billie Cash wrote in a beautiful prayer for me on this blog the other day. 'His journey with you reflects the empty tomb!' Spot on, Billie.

A joyful Easter to you all,

In the fellowship of the easy yoke,
Derick Bingham

P.S. Half an hour after sending in this blog I was called in to the hospital for my second Chemo course.

'Now I want you to know, brothers, that what has happened to me has really served to advance the Gospel. As a result, it has become clear throughout the whole palace guard and to everyone else that I am in chains for Christ. Because of my chains, most of the brothers in the Lord have been encouraged to speak the word of God more courageously and fearlessly'

Written by the Apostle Paul from prison,
Philippians 1:12-14

Monday 4th MAY, 2009
SILVER LININGS AND CLOUDS

Dear everyone,

Warm Greetings. Thank you so much for your continuing kindness in the daily messages that reach me from near and far, wishing me well and assuring me of your prayers. And there's more! My friend Neil Shawcross,[23] the artist, rang to say we would go to the United States on holiday together on the very next day to the day I indicated I wanted to go! The pact, once suggested by me, is that on such a holiday he won't paint and I won't preach! We first met on a flight to New York where he was going to Long Island to paint a portrait of the jazz trumpeter Dizzy Gillespie, and I was heading to Toronto to speak at a Bible Conference. I just love his very memorable paintings of labels of United States Supermarket goods in Café Conor, Stranmillis Road, Belfast. It surely would be quite a holiday, would it not?

I was also cheered greatly the other day when an eight-year-old girl sent me a drawing of the Resurrection, accompanied with the musical notes and words of a little chorus on the same subject. She told me she was praying for

23. Associate of the Royal Ulster Academy, Neil is primarily a portrait painter. He was a lecturer at the Belfast College of Art from 1962 until his retirement in 2004. He has also lectured at Pennsylvania State University. As a friend of mine puts it-'When Neil walks into a room, it lights up!' My favourite Shawcross work is his poignant portrait of the Auschwitz survivor, Dr Helen Lewis. Helen has been a dance choreographer at the Grand Opera House in Belfast. Ironically she was brought in from breaking up roads in a near-death situation at Auschwitz by a brutal female camp Commandant. She ordered her to be involved in choreography at the Christmas party at Auschwitz. It saved her from the gas chamber. She is one of the most amazing people I have ever been privileged to talk with in–depth.

me at home and at Sunday school, and added that she had done the drawing 'all by myself'. I was honoured to receive it.

Another friend and her husband bought me the most expensive set of headphones I have ever had in my life, crafted by Bang and Olufsen (a shop I always drove by)! Now I can really, really listen to my favourite radio programme – Melvyn Bragg's Radio 4 'In our Time' (Thursday morning 9.00-9.45 a.m. and repeated 9.30 to 10.00 p.m.). I so enjoy Melvyn's blog, to which I am signed up weekly.

Two other friends sent me the most exquisite Papuro Italian leather-bound notebook, in which I wrote the first draft of my first blog – its aroma is truly something else. My men Weight Watchers class also sent me a fantastic basket of fruit, and some Ferrero Rocher. A good balanced diet, don't you think?! Eamonn Mallie[24] sent me the entire CD set of Seamus Heaney reading his collected poems. All of these, and wonderfully numerous more kindnesses, brighten long, long days of waiting as Chemo does its work in seeking to treat my Leukaemia - never to speak of the constant kindness and care of the staff of Ward 10 at the Belfast City Hospital. If churches were as united as this hospital staff are at every level of their calling, Northern Ireland and the wider world would soon feel the benefit. They back each other up, they stay within their various disciplines, they minister with the same commitment to all under their care, they show constant diplomacy with awkward patients, and they do their work cheerfully and with studied, incredible patience. To boot, one of the cleaners in my ward, Raphael from Poland who did a degree in Economics at University and became a banker, gave up his profession, he tells me, because he reckoned happiness was not to be found in merely making money. An interesting chap to talk to is Raphael!

---

24. Author and broadcaster specializing in Politics, Security and 20th Century Art.

The experience of having Chemo has a huge effect on one's energy levels. One day one can be feeling very energetic, and the next day even turning a page or holding a conversation is a huge effort. As day follows day and week follows week, I go up and down in spirit through a labyrinth of rising and plunging emotions.

The other night, in the midst of all this, an auxiliary nurse handed me a letter, which had come for me to the hospital. The correspondent pointed out that I did not know her and had never met her personally, but ministry I had given in the past had been graciously used by the Lord to touch her life. She was sure that the Lord was commanding her to pass on to me the words of Jeremiah 29: 11 'For I know I have plans for you', declares the Lord, 'plans to prosper you and not to harm you, plans to give you hope and a future.' Earthly 'hope' and a 'future' are not words freely and unconditionally applied to my condition by the medical profession – believe me! Such words, if given, are given with understandable constraint, and are often accompanied with statistics that run one's mind into an earthly cul-de-sac to say the least. But then, but then, but then……WHAT?

But then, I read the words of Charles Swindoll on the subject of healing. 'It's been my experience', he writes, 'that when God is involved, anything can happen. The one who directed that stone in between Goliath's eyes and split the Red Sea down the middle and leveled that wall around Jericho and brought His Son back from beyond takes delight in mixing up the odds and HE ALTERS THE INEVITABLE AND BYPASSES THE IMPOSSIBLE. The blind songwriter Fanny Crosby put it another way: "chords that were broken will vibrate once more."'[25]

25. Charles Swindoll, The Tale of the Tardy Oxcart , Word Publishing (1998)

I recall a certain time in the past when I preached a series over many weeks on the book of Job. 'I'm coming for the first two chapters' said a lady, 'and the last two, but not all those chapters in the middle!' Ah! All those chapters in the middle. They are, as few others, full of rising and plunging emotions, as Job tried to 'impose meaning' on the incredibly awful circumstances that had over taken him. The important thing, though, is that he did 'impose meaning' on his circumstances. He held tenaciously through all of his suffering that we are not in a meaningless universe, simply at the mercy of some virus or circumstance. That did not mean, though, that he did not have hugely oscillating emotions. He proved, though, that a person can still have a deep affection for God even though there is no immediate evidence of God's love and providence in his or her immediate circumstances.

While in hospital over these many weeks, I have been dipping in to G.M. Ella's biography of William Cowper, one of English literatures most memorable poets.[26] Who in the history of the Christian faith in the Western world experienced the gamut of rising and falling emotions more than Cowper? Son of the King's Chaplain, educated at Westminster School, called to the Bar in 1734, he began to suffer from mental illness under the stress of a public examination, before taking up a post in the House of Lords. He tried to commit suicide with a pair of knitting needles, trying to plunge them into his heart. He then entered an asylum under the care of a doctor who was a Christian, and was converted to Christ through reading Romans 3: 25. Cowper was to suffer from nightmares for the rest of his life, once being out of his mind for six very long months.

Uniquely though, as a writer, he could always write of his emotions when he returned to sanity or from bouts of depression. He 'imposed meaning' on all

26. G.M. Ella, 'William Cowper: Poet of Paradise,' Evangelical Press,1993

he suffered. Where are more poignant lines in all English Literature for anyone who is going through suffering yet, who, at the same time, held the Saviour's sufferings in awe, than these lines of Cowper's?

'Ah! Were I buffeted all day,
Mock'd, crown'd with thorns, and spit upon;
I yet should have no right to say,
My great distress is mine alone.

Let me not angrily declare,
No pain was ever sharp like mine;
Nor murmur at the cross I bear,
But rather weep remembering Thine.'

On the first day of January 1773, Cowper was walking over Olney fields in Buckinghamshire, when he received a sudden premonition that a time of darkness and depression was about to fall on him. Turning to the Lord in his distress, he struggled home and wrote down what he believed, before he went down into what turned out to be a time of very deep darkness. His poem carried some of the most famous lines ever written. Did he 'impose meaning' on his suffering? And how! He wrote:

God moves in a mysterious way,
His wonders to perform,
He plants His footsteps on the sea,
And rides upon the storm.

Deep in unfathomable mines,
Of never failing skill,
He treasures up His bright designs,
And works His sovereign will.

His purposes will ripen fast,
Unfolding every hour,
The bud may have a bitter taste,
But wait, to smell the flower.

Two weeks later, Cowper's friend, the Rev. John Newton who also lived at Olney, wrote of Cowper's condition in his diary: 'I can hardly conceive that anyone in a state of grace and favour with God can be in greater distress; and yet no one waited more clearly with Him, or was more simply devoted to Him in all things.'

I have also been reading Philippians chapter 1, where I find those stirring words of Paul written while in Roman chains. 'Now I want you to know, brothers, that what has happened to me has really served to advance the Gospel.' Did Paul 'impose meaning' in all he had gone through, including severe beatings, shipwreck, heartless criticism and imprisonment? He certainly did.

I stood by the coliseum in Rome last year, and the guide explained that an Imperial Decree had brought the whole ghastly lifestyle that went on there to an end through the influence of Christianity. Such an outcome would have been deemed impossible by millions when the suffering and much despised Paul first entered Rome under arrest so many years previously. There was meaning in it all.

So, if a sparrow does not fall to the ground without the knowledge of my Heavenly Father neither do I.[27] I believe in the power of one. Really? Of course.

In 1645, one vote gave Oliver Cromwell control of England.

In 1649, one vote caused Charles I of England to be executed.

In 1845, one vote brought Texas into the Union.

In 1868, one vote saved President Andrew Johnson from impeachment.

In 1875, one vote changed France from a Monarchy into a Republic.

In 1876, one vote gave R.B. Hayes the United States Presidency.

In 1923, one vote gave Adolf Hitler control of the Nazi party.

If one vote can make such a difference in human history, how much more a life lived for Jesus Christ? Even an hour lived for Him is of inestimable value. And if death or the Lord come?[28] Then there is an eternity to live for Christ, only then it will be far better for it will be service with an unsinning heart.

'Dare you see a Soul at the White Heat?' asked Emily Dickinson.[29] Yes, I see my soul at the White Heat at the moment, and it is a soul with infinite 'hope' and a 'future' beyond calculation in Christ.

Encouraged,
Derick Bingham

27. Luke 10:29-31

28. I Thessalonians 4:14-18

29. Emily Dickinson, American poet (1830-86). From Complete Poems, Little, Brown and Co.,1924. Part One: Life XXX111

'For Christians this pace of change represents an opportunity.
When so much is in flux, when limitless amounts of information,
much of it ephemeral, are instantly accessible on demand, there is
a renewed hunger for that which endures and gives meaning.

The Christian church can speak uniquely to that need, for at the
heart of our faith stands the conviction that all people,
irrespective of race, background or circumstance, can find lasting
significance and purpose in the Gospel of Jesus Christ.'

Her Majesty, Queen Elizabeth II
Speaking at the opening of the Church of England Synod 2005.

Thursday 4th JUNE, 2009
A MESSAGE FROM THE HOUSE OF LORDS

Dear everyone,

From the midst of the present crisis in the Parliament of the United Kingdom, a Peer in the House of Lords - for whom I have the very highest regard - most kindly emailed me to encourage me in my present storm of Leukaemia. He shared the following statement 'we live in sad and difficult times. The Scripture in my mind is "Them that honour me I will honour and they that despise me shall be lightly esteemed".'[30] The Scripture quoted from the first book of Samuel was like an arrow in a sure place – I was deeply challenged by it. We often quote the first part of the Scripture but seldom the last part.

It all got me thinking about a former time in Westminster Hall, sitting early one morning with the former Speaker of the House of Commons, Michael Martin[31] chatting to him at the National Prayer Breakfast.[32] There too sat Anne Graham Lotz, the daughter of Dr. Billy Graham and National Prayer Breakfast speaker for that morning. 'Did you attend Dr. Graham's meetings at the Kelvin Hall in Glasgow?' I asked Mr. Martin, gently. "I was only a wee boy then", he replied, "but a fellow metal worker called Jack Mitchell went forward at one of those meetings, and subsequently went into the Christian ministry", he said.

"It was good seed, your father sowed 50 years ago, wasn't it?" I said to Anne Graham. I mused in my heart at how that seed had surfaced 50 years later in our discussion of the spiritual life of Jack Mitchell, in the hall where Kings and Queens of the United Kingdom lie in state. The potent power of the seed of the Word of God is actually, when you muse on it, eternal in its

---

30. I Samuel 2:30
31. Now Baron Martin of Springburn
32. I was a guest of the Rt. Hon Jeffrey Donaldson who gently lowered me into the middle of it all! Jeffrey was that year's Chairman.

influence, never to speak of 50 years. So, sow it, Christian, sow it. Don't go through your day without scattering some of it in the corners only you can reach.

The Deputy Foreign Minister of Israel also turned up for breakfast at the same table that morning, along with his bodyguards. He had his kosher breakfast food wrapped in cling film. He was a Rabbi and asked a very surprised Anne Graham Lotz if he could borrow her Bible. He started thumbing through it, obviously looking for something. I wondered if that was what a Rabbi did at that time of the morning but, no, it subsequently turned out that he too was to be a speaker that morning. He got up and addressed us from the life of Abraham, reading from Anne's Bible! All in all it was truly a most memorable breakfast.

At an extraordinary gathering near Windsor in 1215, a famous document emerged known as Magna Carta. King John signed it under force, and it allowed for the formation of a powerful Parliament. It was the first written document expounding democracy on these Islands. Now that very democracy to which the Magna Carta gave birth is under threat by the current expenses scandal in Parliament.

Having preached across South Korea, where Margaret and I had to make sure we were indoors by curfew time, lest we ended up in prison, I have a deep interest in news from the Korean Peninsula. In Seoul, the main thoroughfare can be turned into a fighter jet runway in minutes. Will they have to do that soon? God forbid. Continuing terrorist threats and atrocities across the world brings international fear into millions of hearts.

Our times are truly disturbing times. Powerfully, a poem has been surfacing in my mind during the current moral crisis in these Islands. It is by William Wordsworth, and I learnt it at school. It is worth meditating on:-

Milton! Thou shouldst be living at this hour:
England hath need of thee: she is a fen
Of stagnant waters: altar, sword, and pen,
Fireside, the heroic wealth of hall and bower,
Have forfeited their ancient English dower
Of inward happiness. We are selfish men;
Oh! Raise us up, return to us again;
And give us manners, virtue, freedom, power
Thy soul was like a Star, and dwelt apart;
Thou hadst a voice whose sound was like the sea:
Pure as the naked heavens, majestic, free,
So didst thou travel on life's common way,
In cheerful godliness; and yet thy heart
The lowliest duties on herself did lay.[33]

Wordsworth obviously turned to Milton's life and work for inspiration at a time when he felt everything in national and domestic life was becoming 'a fen of stagnant waters.' When the godly peer sent me the Scripture on his mind, it sent me to read the life of Samuel again, from which the Scripture comes. I found inspiration there at this disturbing time.

When you think about it, the story began with suffering. Samuel's mother had been barren for 'the Lord had closed her womb'. She became the object of the most unbelievable cruelty. A 'rival', we are told, provoked her. I take it that the 'rival' was a fellow Israelite, for 'whenever Hannah went up to the house of the Lord, her rival provoked her till she wept and would not eat'. Is it not amazing who the Devil gets to do his work for him?

33. London, 1802, Sonnet ccxiii

Think, though, of the religious hypocrisy around Hannah, and the corruption of Israel's national life. It included the gross sexual behavior of Eli's sons, and the women of Israel who were implicit in it. Priests were at that time taking more than their fair share of meat sacrifices brought by the people to the Lord in their worship. God accused Eli, the High Priest: 'why do you scorn my sacrifice and offering that I prescribed for my dwelling? Why do you honour your sons more than Me by fattening yourselves on the choice parts of every offering made by my people Israel?'

In the very heart of all this corruption Hannah, the Scriptures say, 'stood up.' I love those two words! (Who, in our nation, is going to 'stand up'?) She had had enough. She decided to go to the temple of the Lord at Shiloh (the tabernacle, as it was then) and pray to the Lord about her problem. When she got there the High Priest was so far away from the Lord that he did not know the difference between a praying woman and a drunken one. 'How long will you keep on getting drunk?', he accused her. If any person had the right to walk out of a place of worship and wash her hands of the whole thing, Hannah measured into such a right. To her eternal credit she stood firm, and looking into the face of that lazy, miserable priest of Israel she said 'Not so, my lord.' Here was a woman who was prepared to stand up to the most powerfully positioned spiritual leader in Israel and not let his position, power, or insults divert her from the truth. How did she do it? Well, as the poet put it:

'Faith came singing into my room;
Other guests took flight.
Fear and anxiety, grief and gloom,
Sped out into the night.

And I wondered how such peace could be,
Faith said gently, 'Don't you see?'
They really could not live with me!' [34]

How different things would have been had Hannah reacted naturally. As it happened, she reacted spiritually. By faith, she asked the Lord for a son. And when he came, God shared state secrets with him while he was still in his boyhood. Think about it: God shared state secrets with a boy. Even Eli, on the third occasion we are told, suddenly 'realized that the Lord was calling the boy.' We read: 'the Lord was with Samuel as he grew up, and let none of his words fall to the ground. And all Israel from Dan to Beersheba recognized that Samuel was attested as a prophet of the Lord. The Lord continued to appear at Shiloh, and there He revealed himself to Samuel through His word.'

Think of it: God bypassed the clever, the rich, the influential, the many ranks of Israel's leaders in 'altar, sword and pen' and shared His mind, heart, and intentions with a child, and used him to turn a nation around. God can still speak to a child and use that child to turn a nation around: even your child in your nation or children under your spiritual influence. Be encouraged.

Did Samuel's mother ever realize that her son would one day judge Israel from the town he originally came from - from his mother's hometown? 'Samuel', says Scripture, 'continued as judge over Israel all the days of his life. From year to year he went on a circuit from Bethel to Gilgal to Mizpah, judging Israel in all those places. But he always went back to Ramah, where his home was, and there he also judged Israel and he built an altar there to the Lord.' In

34. Poem by Elizabeth Anderson (1927-2001). Her husband Bill kindly gave me permission to use it. He tells me that he found his wife's poem scribbled on a scrap of paper amongst cooking recipes. For more of her poems see www.bettyspoety.co.uk

truth, under God, Samuel became the kingmaker in Israel. He eventually anointed David as king, from whose descendants the Messiah came, in whom our hope and destiny is placed. It all began, though, with Hannah's tears and her amazing spiritual reaction to her suffering.

Dr. M.R. De Haan once calculated that if all the tears shed in the world could be barreled and poured into a canal, such a waterway would stretch from New York to San Francisco. He maintained that it would make a river in which barges could be floated. Few would doubt him.

You and I may be near the point of despair at times, and although we profess to know God in Christ, our adversary comes like Job's wife and says, 'Curse God and die.' Let us do no such thing. Let us not be diverted. We remember in the dark what God has taught us in the light. We press on with the work that lies at our hand, inspired by the fact that God literally changed history through a broken hearted, childless, sorely provoked Hannah. He can do the same through us, if we let Him.[35]

As for me, I can't go to a church service at the moment because of the risk of infection. I do miss the fellowship of fellow Christians. I have had spelled out to me the nature of the cancer in my blood, which though currently in remission, can return exceedingly swiftly and aggressively. I have also had spelled out to me the side effects I can expect from the Chemo drug I will be given by injection beginning on June 8th. But then I read Hannah's words, coming out of her experience:

---

35. For an amazing modern story on this theme have a look at The Washington Post article online entitled 'The Pastor who has Obama's attention' (Oct 14th 2009). That Pastor's mother is my writing colleague Billie Cash who has written some beautiful prayers for me and my family on my blog throughout my illness. Her new book on prayer entitled 'The Shelter,' published this Fall by Ambassador International, is a winner.

'My heart rejoices in the Lord;
In the Lord my strength is lifted high…..
There is no one holy like the Lord;
There is no one besides You;
There is no Rock like our God…..
He raises the poor from the dust
And lifts the needy from the ash heap
He seats them with princes and has them
Inherit a throne of honour …..
He will guard the feet of the saints.'

Hannah's song makes my spirit lift, and the truth it expounds steadies my mind and heart in my leukaemic storm. One thing clearly shines out from the story of Hannah and Samuel: beautiful things can emerge out of suffering. Even mine. I am so grateful that a Peer in the House of Lords took time to send me that wee verse from the first book of Samuel.

Onward!
Derick Bingham

*-A letter reminding me of one of the most moving
moments of my life-*

*I received the following most kind letter during my present illness from Tom and
Doreen Lewis of BEE International. It highlights a deeply memorable moment
while I was ministering God's Word in Arad, Romania. Tom and Doreen are
involved internationally in a ministry known as Bible Education by Extension.
This is a ministry that provides seminary level Bible training to pastors and
church leadership who have no access to Biblical training. Most of these
leaders live in restricted access countries. This ministry's vision is to provide
access to Biblical training to anyone who desires to mature as a disciple of
Jesus Christ. See www.beeworld.org*

My Dear Derick,

I have just returned from the United States. I was speaking at a large
Missions conference in Memphis - First Evangelical Church Memphis - when
Doreen informed me of your illness. I was shocked and deeply saddened to
hear of your illness and asked the church to pray which they did – fervently -
for you, Margaret and the girls.

We continue to think and pray for you every day. You have been such a
good friend to me and BEE international. I remember with joy our time together
in Romania shortly after the revolution. Do you remember the time in
Bucharest when we visited the Palace of Ceausescu and the new government
buildings, which were never occupied by the Communists? Then walking down
the Boulevard of the Revolution our attention focused as our ears caught the

strains of the children's chorus 'Our God is so good, so great and so mighty there's nothing our God cannot do.' We entered the building to be met by one of my former students and octogenarian, Carman. He had taken over one of Ceausescu's apartments and turned it into a Christian bookshop and publishing house. What a great time we had with that dear aging servant of God!

You recounted that incident in Arad a few days later in the Sunday afternoon service in Maranatha Baptist Church when almost 3,000 had gathered to hear you speak. You were speaking on Queen Esther, Mordecai and the conspiracy of Haman against Mordecai. The Lord turned the tables on Haman and he perished instead. You then shared the incident in Bucharest with Carman drawing a comparison with Ceausescu and Haman. The whole congregation began to cry including your translator Pastor Doru Popa. When you had finished speaking no one moved - the Maranatha congregation should have left to make room for the next service due to be conducted in the same building! As you were to speak at the second service you ended up with two congregations in the one building with over half having to listen from the street outside! You said afterwards that it was an incredible moment and a highlight of your ministry! It was for both of us.

The Lord has blessed your ministry over many years Derick and it has been a joy and privilege to have ministered with you and to have you as a friend.

Be assured of our continued prayers as you go through this battle. You are loved in Christ.

Your friends,
Tom and Doreen

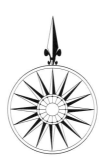

Tuesday 30th JUNE, 2009
BEING IN A SPACIOUS PLACE

Dear everyone,

Warm greetings. I am truly staggered and humbled by the fact that virtually every time I go out on the street, round and about the city in which I live and in the surrounding countryside, people tell me they are reading my blog – my letters on the Net. Amazingly, it has slipped out across the world too. Thank you all for your interest, prayers and concern and the continuing, motivating, kindly, well-wishing mail I am receiving.[36]

It is good to report that last Tuesday (June 23rd), as I received a check-up on my condition at the hospital, I was told that the medical team are pleased with my progress. I even heard the word 'great' being used. I am grateful, believe me. My blood counts have remained acceptable following the daily injections of the 'new' Chemo drug over five days.

The next round of injections begins on July 20th, God willing. I am being brought in as an outpatient every Tuesday to have my blood counts taken, which monitors my reaction to the drug. My heart is, in a way, in my mouth on Tuesdays, but I do try to keep 2 Chronicles 16; 12 in mind. Really? Really. It says:

'In the thirty-ninth year of his reign Asa was afflicted with a disease in his feet. Though his disease was severe, even in his illness he did not seek help from the Lord, but only from the physicians.'

36. Amazingly the Press lifted these letters and the BBC. I then began to get a reaction through hundreds of messages by email, card and letter.

Asa had a history of not relying on the Lord. Earlier in his life a seer called Hanani visited him and pointed out that 'because you relied on the king of Aram and not on the Lord your God, the army of the king of Aram has escaped from your hand….for the eyes of the Lord range throughout the earth to strengthen those whose hearts are fully committed to him. You have done a foolish thing, and from now on you will be at war.' Asa promptly put the seer in prison!

Notice in this story that the Lord did not hold Asa's seeking help from physicians against him. What the Lord objected to was that he had sought help only from that corner. I am in a huge debt to the physicians and nursing staff who have cared for me over the past 122 days. Their skills, patience, counsel and dedication have been deeply appreciated. As a disciple of the Lord Jesus though, I try to keep in mind that ultimately my help comes from the Lord who uses physicians. I also try to keep in mind that the Lord who is my Healer is also my Master. He who gives also has the right to take away. I submit to what he wants.

Two helpful women have touched my life across recent weeks. One of them, a hospital chaplain, the Rev Muriel Cromie, approached my bedside one day and read to me the words of Psalm 31:8b. It is the verse where David acknowledges how the Lord has set his feet in a 'spacious place.' Muriel felt that it was a promise from God to me in my life at this time. A few weeks later Billie Cash, the gifted American writer (see billiecash.com), sent me a message in which she pointed out 'Your suffering has become a "spacious place" in the Spirit (Ps 31b).' One woman lives in Northern Ireland, and the other lives in Tennessee and they do not know each other to my knowledge. They both reckoned that the Lord had put my feet in a 'spacious place.' What does it mean? I sat down by the Lagan river in Belfast in a little coffee shop with my ever-nurturing friend Sir Nigel Hamilton[37] this week, where, in the context of my present circumstances, we discussed the phrase from David's Psalm in depth. I came home and the following meditation emerged.

David was in narrow place, to all intents and purposes, when he wrote Psalm 31b, was he not? In the very same Psalm he wrote that:

1) A trap had been set for him.
2) He was in anguish of soul.
3) His eyes were weak with sorrow, his soul and body with grief.
4) His life was consumed with anguish, his years with groaning.
5) His strength was failing because of affliction.
6) His bones had grown weak.
7) He was held in utter contempt by his neighbours.
8) He was a dread to his friends.
9) When his friends saw him on the street they fled.
10) His friends forgot him as though he were dead.
11) Terror lay on every side of him.
12) He was being slandered.

Is it not fascinating that, despite his narrow circumstances, David maintained that the Lord had planted his feet in a 'spacious place'?

My place at the moment is a narrow circumstance. My medical Professor tells me that I have a 30% chance of living 3-5 years; some weeks back it was

---

37. Sir Nigel Hamilton, KCB, former Head of the Northern Ireland Civil Service (2002-2008), which he joined in 1970. He was made an honorary graduate of the University of Ulster and awarded a Doctorate of the University (2008) in recognition of his contribution to public administration in Northern Ireland especially during the years of the Northern Ireland peace process. His friendship has been a tower of strength to me both before and during this present illness. He is currently Chairman of The Prince's Trust in Northern Ireland and Deputy Lord Lieutenant for the City of Belfast.

said I had a 5% chance of living at all. But the Bible is not into percentages, is it? The Lord knows the day of his coming or our death, and as for life, the same Psalm says 'but I trust in you, O Lord: I say you are my God. My times are in your hands.'

So what have I learned? I have learned that a narrow circumstance can become a spacious place. David lifted his pen, despite his circumstances, and nurtured millions. Really? Of course. He is now published in virtually every language on the face of the earth. In his Psalms there is every variety of human experience and incredible hope. When you are filled with ecstasy or stricken by depression, there is a Psalm for you. When you gain and when you lose, there is a Psalm to pick up your mood. Here is ethics, history and prophecy. Here is talk of the stars and the forbidding desert. Here is sheer delight in God. Here is a mirror into your very soul.

When you think about it, looking across biblical history, Abraham was in a very narrow circumstance when he left Lot to the well-watered plains. Yet the Lord eventually took his childless servant outside one night and said 'Look up at the heavens and count the stars - if indeed you can count them. So shall your offspring be.'[38] A spacious place, or what?

Joseph was in narrow circumstance when he was put in a hole in the ground by his downright wicked brothers and then sold into slavery. As he headed down to Egypt as a slave, what were his thoughts? It surely did not seem to be a path to the governorship of Egypt, the saving of North Africa from starvation and the preservation of the line of the Messiah - but that is just what it was. The narrow was in fact incredibly spacious.[39]

---

38. Genesis 14: 4 - 6

39. Genesis: Chapters 37- 39

Moses was also in very narrow circumstance. He was in an ark of bulrushes, surrounded by crocodiles that were and are the second largest in the world. On the throne was Pharaoh, just as vicious, who would have had Moses slaughtered on the spot if discovered. 'If it is a boy', he had ordered the midwives in Egypt dealing with any Hebrew births, 'kill him.'

The ark of bulrushes in fact turned out to be a very spacious place, because Pharaoh's daughter saw it and had it opened. The future of Israel hung upon a baby's tears. Moses could not have been in a more spacious place, and was raised as the son of Pharaoh's daughter and was schooled in one of the greatest civilizations on earth. He later led two and a half million people out of slavery.[40]

Was not Ruth in a narrow circumstance as she turned into a field near Bethlehem as a gleaner? It was just about the narrowest place she could have been; yet in reality it could not have been more spacious. The field belonged to Boaz, and Boaz belonged to the Lord. They married and their grandson was King David, whose greater son was Christ. He was laid in a manager in the very same town centuries later - the Saviour of the world, and me too!!![41] There was no sign of all this at all when Ruth headed out to glean on that far off morning.

Jonah was in a truly narrow place in terms of future survival - the stomach of a whale. 'The engulfing waters threatened me,' he wrote, 'the deep surrounded me; seaweed was wrapped around my head. To the roots of the mountains I sank down; the earth beneath barred me in forever. But you

---

40. Genesis: Chapters; 1 - 12
41. Ruth Chapters 1 - 4

brought my life up from the pit, O Lord my God.'[42] Jonah was out of the will of God. He was stubborn and a racist, yet he was to see the repentance of the entire city of Nineveh under his preaching. Not much sign of it when the seaweed was wrapped around his head, was there?

And what shall we say about Elijah? He had run away from a scolding woman's tongue and was hiding from his ministry in a cave. But the Lord had set his feet in a spacious place and restored him to his ministry.[43] Elijah's successor - who was given a double portion of his spirit - got up one morning early, and an army with horses and chariots surrounded the city. 'Oh, my Lord, what shall we do?' his servant asked. 'Don't be afraid', the prophet answered, and asked the Lord to open the young man's eyes. The young fellow soon discovered that while his feet were in a narrow place 'the hills were full of horses and chariots of fire all round Elisha.'[44]

As for Job, when very ill with sores from the soles of his feet to the top of his head, bereaved and listening to his wife who, suggesting he was in such a narrow place he would be better to curse God and die, he absolutely refused to do so.[45] And the result? He wrote a book, reckoned by some to be the oldest in the Bible. The book of Job resolutely soars above that narrowest of places, namely, the fear of the grave. Job states that should worms destroy his body, he would in his flesh see God![46] Job became one of the greatest examples of perseverance through suffering in history. Now that is what I call spaciousness.

As for me, though in a narrow place, I have actually found myself, as Muriel and Billie pointed out, in a spacious place. Pray for me across the next

---

42. Jonah 2: 5 - 6
43. I Kings Chapter 19 - 2Kings Chapter2
44. 2Kings 6:15 - 17
45. Job 3:9 - 10
46. Job 19:23 - 27

few weeks, as I am deeply involved in writing a new free booklet with the TBF and KL Thompson Trust. This is to be placed, hopefully, in an extremely strategic place in a great city, abroad. Of all the work I have been privileged to do, I consider the little booklets I have been graciously allowed to write and place with this Trust the most important work in which I have ever been involved.[47] Their reach is awesome in the hand of God. A taxi driver in Dublin recently asked for 1,000 copies of the booklet *A Guinness with a Difference; the Story of the Whistling Ploughboy of Ecclefechan.* He had been a plumber in the Guinness brewery in Dublin (the mind boggles!) and had come to faith in Christ. He has now found a new ministry in giving the booklet to each of his passengers! God bless him, richly.

When I began to recover recently, I was graciously told that if there was anything I ever wished to write, then I would be supported in writing it at this time. The present booklet on which I am currently working is what I have wished to write for years, but the way did not open. I cannot say more at present, but just this. Pray for the placing of this booklet in a very historic place. I will let you know in time what it is all about, as the Lord leads. I sincerely believe that I have never been privileged to write a more strategic piece in evangelism.

Onward!
Derick Bingham

---

47. See tbft.tv

*'I have just heard, to my great surprise, that I have but
a few days to live. It may be that before this reaches you,
I shall have entered the palace. Don't trouble to write.
We shall meet in the morning'*

Written by F.B. Meyer (1847-1929) to a friend a few
days before he died.

(Source; LB Cowman, 1933, Consolation, Los Angeles:
Oriental Missionary Society.)

Wednesday 5th AUGUST, 2009
LOOKING FOR COMFORT

Dear everyone,

Warm greetings. It is soooooooooooo good to report another successful five days of Chemo injections, two per day. They bring down one's energy levels, but they are doing what my medical team call 'consolidating' work. I am deeply grateful. Thank you to all who continually pray for me, including the lady behind the glass at the Post Office, who told me so a few minutes ago. Her church has a prayer chain and the person who liaises it all rang her up and said:

'You probably won't know this person but…'

'Oh I know him', said the ever-encouraging 'post mistress' who has processed the mail I have given her over many years.

Such moments, even in a Post Office, are God moments. 'It was not your time yet', she said with a comforting smile, as she pointed out that the Lord must still have something for me to do. As it happened, I had just handed her a package that contained the current text of a new booklet I have written, thus sending it on its way to Ross Wilson, the sculptor and artist who has just powerfully portrayed my subject for this booklet. I plead further prevailing prayer for this work, as it is now at a very sensitive stage for placing in a great strategic city abroad. My daughter Kerrie is hard at work in imaging it, and her gift flourishes. When I am eventually able to tell you, God willing, the awesome timing of it all, you will know what Ross means when he says as these occasions surface, 'You'd almost think someone arranged it'! For sure.

Speaking of comforting things, I was at the Cancer Centre at the City Hospital recently, and it was great to further talk in-depth with Dr. Andrew Drain who has the same illness as I have. He is a deep inspiration with his shining faith. We encouraged one another in the Lord our God. My unforgettable image of Andrew is of him heading out of the Cancer Centre one day several months ago, following his hospital appointment, with his laptop under his arm, going to preach in Ballymena on the subject of Job! He has no idea how that courageous action comforted me and, no doubt, his listeners. Mr. Faithful, I'd call him.

Comfort is a wonderful thing. 'Can a mother forget the baby at her breast?' asks Scripture, 'and have no compassion on the child she has borne?' The answer to the question is that, yes, some mothers have actually done that. But, says the same Scripture of the Lord, 'though she may forget, I will not forget you. See, I have engraved you on the palms of my hands.'[48]

As I have read and listened to the huge debate raging in the nation at the moment about assisted suicide, the answer is found in this verse. Why would I deliberately take my own life with my own hands, or ask others to assist me in such an action, when the Lord's mighty hands are engraved with my name on them? Those hands can take me across the River of Death to the land where there flows the River of Life, as clear as crystal, where the leaves of the Tree of Life are for the healing of the nations. There the throne of God and of the Lamb stands and his servants will serve Him. There they will see His face and His name will be on their foreheads. There will be no more night. They will not need the light of a lamp or the light of the sun, for the Lord God will give them light. And they will reign forever and ever.[49]

48. Isaiah 49:15-16
49. Rev 22:1- 5

What is brave and honourable about deliberately taking one's own life out of those divine hands into one's own hands? There is nothing brave and honourable about it whatsoever. I did not choose to be born; God gave the burden of life to me through my parents. So it is with my death or rapture.

'Think it not strange, child of God', writes the great F.B.Meyer in his magnificent late 19th- early 20th Century writing style, 'concerning the fiery trial that tries thee, as though some strange thing had happened. Rejoice! For it is a sure sign that thou art on the right track. If in an unknown country, I am informed that I must pass through a valley where the sun is hidden, or over a stony bit of road, to reach my abiding place when I come to it, each moment of shadow or jolt of the carriage tells me that I am on the right road. So when a child of God passes through affliction he is not surprised.'[50]

A couple of years ago in Bournemouth, a kind friend of mine called George Willcock enquired for me as to the burial plot number of F.B.Meyer, as I wanted to visit it to pay homage to one of the greatest spiritual writers I have ever come across, and to whom I owe an enormous debt. We searched long and hard in the huge graveyard but could not find the plot. There is not even a headstone to mark the burial place of the great spiritual giant who preached at the Keswick Convention one night on holiness and the local Post Office ran out of postal orders the next day because Christians were paying their bills!!! That's what I call preaching. The man whose books sold by the million, and was read by factory workers and royalty alike in his day, has not even got a memorial raised to him on earth. No matter, his reward in the Celestial city truly far outweighs any earthly memorial.

'Look out for comfort', writes Meyer in his classic (and I mean classic) work 'Christ in Isaiah', 'it will come *certainly*. Wherever the nettle grows, beside

50. Christ in Isaiah: Chapter 1 "Comfort Ye, Comfort Ye' (Marshall, Morgan and Scott, Ltd London, 1950). One of the greatest books I have ever read.

it grows the dock-leaf; and wherever there is severe trial, there is, somewhere at hand, a sufficient store of comfort, though our eyes, like Hagar's, are often holden that we cannot see it. But it is a sure as the faithfulness of God. "I never had" says Bunyan, writing of his twelve years of imprisonment, "in all my life, so great an insight into the Word of God as now; insomuch that I have often said, were it lawful, I could pray for greater trouble, for the greater comfort's sake." God cannot forget his child. He cannot leave us to suffer, unsuccoured and alone. He runs to meet the prodigal; but he rides on a cherub, and he flies on the wings of the wind to the sinking disciple.'

Meyer adds, mark it well, that comfort will come proportionately. 'Thy Father holds a pair of scales. This on the right is called As, and is for thine afflictions; this on the left is called So, and is for thy comforts. And the beam is always kept level. The more the trial, the more thy comfort. As the sufferings of Christ abound in us, so our consolation also aboundeth through Christ.'

As if this were not enormously enough, our comfort, Meyer states, will come *Divinely*. He points out that if one were meeting a friend at the railway terminus, it is better to know by what route to expect him, lest the friend arrive on one platform while we await him on another. So it is with comfort. We do not look to man, ultimately, for comfort, 'for he cannot reach low enough into the heart.' Shall we look to angels? 'No; among the many ministries that God entrusts to them, He seldom sends them to comfort; perhaps they are too strong, or they have never suffered. To bind up a broken heart requires a delicacy of touch even Gabriel has not. God preserves to Himself the prerogative of comfort. It is a Divine art. The choice name of the Son and the Spirit is *Paraclete* (the Consoler or Comforter). Thine is the God of all comfort.'

Comfort also comes *mediately* and *variously*. Mediately our comfort abounds through Christ. Variously it may come through a letter, a card, or even a bunch of grapes etc.

What do we do, then, with this comfort? Store it up. Keep a record in your heart and mind, or even in your journal, of the ways in which God comforts you. It will 'divert thy thoughts from thy miseries to the outnumbering mercies: and it will take away that sense of useless and aimless existence, which is often the sufferer's weariest cross.'

Finally, Meyer urges us to pass on the comfort we receive. He tells how a kind-hearted man found a schoolboy crying, because the latter had not got quite enough to pay his fare home. Suddenly, he remembered how, many years before, he had been in the same plight, but had been helped by an unknown friend, who enjoined him some day to pass the kindness on. Now he saw that the anticipated moment had arrived. He took the weeping boy aside, told him the story, paid his fare, and asked him, in his turn, to pass the kindness on. And as the train moved from the station, the lad cried cheerily, 'I will pass it on, sir.' So that act of wonderful love in being passed on through the world, nor will it stay till its ripples have circled the globe and meet again.' Selah.

How heartbreaking it was when we, as a family, lost my Uncle Wesley when he was killed by a runaway horse at the Castlewellan Show last month. Our prayer is that his daughter Hazel, her husband Peter and their son Samuel will know the comfort I have just written about. It is comforting to know that my Uncle has gone to that city where he will no longer live by faith, but will live by sight. And what a sight!

Thanks again to the multitude of you who have prayed for me. I will let you know how things progress across the coming weeks in the good and perfect will of God.

In the fellowship of the easy yoke,
Derick Bingham

' Suffering purges. Suffering positions. Suffering prepares. Weaned again … we become more alive to His Words and Worth. Being graven in His hands is the place of deepest assurance. His hands are fruitful, blessed, faithful and that is where you are, my friend. Prayer for you is encircling the globe. How amazing is prayer! With irony; not only does God bid us to lift and strengthen another but in the process we who pray are being changed the most…. for God is partnering with us. As we pray for you we also are progressing toward a more complete Life in Him, one that is intentional and abiding. Your illness is changing us. Awesome! Miraculous! Transcendent! Sending prayer for your continued healing and blessing to you both in Jesus Name. "Though the mountains be shaken and the hills removed, yet my love for you will not be shaken nor my covenant of peace be removed, says the Lord who has compassion on you." Isaiah 54:4. Standing on the promises we advance.'

A prayer received from Billie Cash on 1st September 2009.

Wednesday 23rd SEPTEMBER, 2009
THE MAN FROM AUGHLISNAFIN

Dear everyone,

Warm Greetings. I want to emphasise to you all that the effectual, fervent prayers of so many on my behalf continues to bring me inestimable comfort. Thank you all so much. I now move on from another round of the new Chemo drug and my condition remains stable.

I truthfully report that I have known a very deep, indefinable joy as I face the unknown. I realize the seriousness of my condition and do not write lightly of it. But the joy of the Lord is very real to me. I do tire easily and am seeking only to do those things that my strength allows. Writing is particularly my open door, and I am going through it as the Lord leads me. More of that soon.

In the meantime I thought I would pass on to you my tribute to my Uncle Wesley who was killed by a runaway horse at Castlewellan Show, back in July. I trust it will encourage those of you who teach young people the things of God, because they go deeper than we think.

Millions of us remember Alistair Cooke, who in his lifetime became a broadcasting legend. His famous 'Letter from America' presented all that was best about the country he eventually chose to live in. I counted his broadcasts one of life's treasures. His was an achievement that has never been matched. Alistair lived into his nineties. He spoke of God being nothing more than 'a consoling myth' but also admitted that he could be wrong. His wife Jane would demand to know of her daughter Susie, who became a Congregational minister, "How can you believe in God and science?" "How can you not?" Susie replied.

Alistair gradually transmuted into Susie's most enthusiastic promoter. Did he, she wondered, envy her the certainty of her faith? 'He told me once,' she said, 'that hardly a day went by without his remembering a verse of Scripture that he learned at the age of eleven or twelve.' Who but God knows how that verse was used in Alistair's life as he faced eternity?[51]

A Tribute to my Uncle

Our family has farmed in Aughlisnafin for over two centuries and nobody ever epitomized life in this hidden and beautiful area of South Down around the Moneycarragh River better than my Uncle Wesley. As children we used to play in his flax dam, make tunnels in the bales of hay in his barn and swing on the best rope swing on the island of Ireland that hung enticingly from a branch in the huge oak tree in his yard. We chased mice amid the stooks at harvest time, as he made sure the huge belt of the old orange painted harvester did not entangle us. And how we loved it when the lemonade man would drive his van up the long lane and Uncle Wesley would stock up. We always maintained that Hazel, his daughter, was weaned on white lemonade!

Living in his home before electricity came to Aughlisnafin, while my parents built a new home in Newcastle, how well I remember going to bed up the narrow stairs, holding a candle that made memorable shadows on the little bedroom wall. I remember the damson tree outside the window and Uncle Wesley's vine that he nurtured in his greenhouse, and the taste of the grapes that flourished there. I often

---

51. Nick Clarke, 'Alistair Cooke, The Biography', Wiedenfield and Nicolson, 1999.

sat proudly on the mudguard of his grey Ferguson tractor as he carefully ploughed his fields, as flocks of birds followed us. One of Uncle Wesley's heroes was Harry Ferguson of Dromara and his incredible engineering feats that changed the face of agriculture around the world.

Family Christmas's at his home were something else. The table groaned with delicious food, because his sisters Lily and Ruth and his sister-in-law, Eleanor and his wife Elizabeth were among the best cooks in the land. And every year we played Uncle Wesley's most famous game. It was memory game and it was also played whenever a crowd of visitors went to his home for any kind of major gathering! It was called 'A good fat hen and about she goes!' This was the first line that must be repeated with all the others that followed without mistake or you were out!

A good fat hen and about she goes... he would say... then came ...
... two ducks. ..a good fat hen and about she goes... and then ...
three grey screeching wild geese...two ducks...a good fat hen and about she goes etc .

When visitors arrived at... *four flat bottomed fly boats flying up the lake of Genesarret* or... *six Anti-Deluvian Patriarchs with their beards well dipped in the gold of Ophar*, we split our sides laughing at attempts people made to pronounce it all. I have seldom seen as much innocent laughter in my life!

Uncle Wesley was famous for his humour. If he were flying with a Hedley Murphy tour of Israel, there he would be in the heart of it all with his jokes and stories. If he was at a wedding, or wherever he was, he was sure to be found in some corner, surrounded by happy people.

But although full of fun, he had his serious side. He did not shirk the call of the Gospel, the best news in the world, and he became a follower and disciple of Jesus Christ. As children we remember him at the Sunday School at Ballywillwill Gospel Hall leading the singing. He taught us of a cleansing fountain deep and wide, of the wise man who built his house upon the rock, and I can still hear him sing,

'She lost it; she lost it,
That little piece of silver,
She sought it, she sought it,
Wherever could it be?
Under the carpet, down by the door,
Into the cupboard,
All over the floor,
Until she found it, she found it,
How happy she would be,
How happy are the children who are found by thee.'

Nothing brought him greater pleasure than seeing young people trust Christ as their Saviour and Lord.

He remained deeply faithful to the Lord Jesus, and supported all those who preached the Gospel wherever they were found. No sectarian spirit ever dominated his Christian witness.

He had a particular skin growth in his hand, and when he went to the Royal Victoria Hospital in Belfast the surgeon asked him if he had any connection with the Vikings. It seems they had the same growth in their hands. Fascinatingly, a few years later, a member of the

McNeill family in New Zealand was tracing the genealogy of the family and asked Uncle Wesley for a DNA sample. He gladly gave it. Incredibly it established that he was part of an unbroken male line to the Vikings! That certainly proves that our family were not always Unionists or Evangelicals! I always maintain that he had the bluest eyes you ever saw, inherited by my daughter Claire - proving their Scandanavian origins!

Just last Wednesday, my Uncle Wesley rang me up on the phone. He was very courageously fighting cancer and was deeply concerned about mine. It was obvious from his conversation that life since Aunt Elizabeth's death had proved extremely lonely for him because they were deeply devoted to one another. The Scripture says that 'we know not what a day may bring forth' and Uncle Wesley's heartbreaking and tragic death has totally stunned us all, far and wide. I am sure, though, that as he crossed the River of Death the words of Mr. Stand Fast from The Pilgrim's Progress are more than apt:

'I see myself', said Stand Fast, *'now at the end of my journey, my toilsome days are ended. I am going to see that head that was crowned with thorns, and that face that was spat upon for me. I have formerly lived by hearsay and faith but now go where I shall live by sight and shall be with Him in whose company I delight myself. I have loved to hear my Lord spoken of; and wherever I have seen the print of His shoe in the earth, there I have coveted to set my foot too. His name to me has been as a perfume-box; yea, sweeter than all perfume. His voice to me has been most sweet; and His countenance*

I have more desired than they that have most desired the light of the sun. His word I did use to gather my food, and for antidotes against my fainting. He has held me, and hath kept me form mine iniquities; yea, my steps hath he strengthened in his way.'

'Glorious it was to see,' says Bunyan, 'how the open region was filled with singers and players on stringed instruments, to welcome the Pilgrims as they went up, and followed one another in at the beautiful gate of the city.' [52]

Uncle Wesley has left a legacy that will linger as long as Aughlisnafin remains and as for him, he has gone to his eternal reward.

In the fellowship of the easy yoke,
Derick Bingham

---

52. John Bunyan,' The Pilgrim's Progress,' Part 2, Section X, 1678

There Is a Hope

There is a hope that burns within my heart,
That gives me strength for every passing day;
A glimpse of glory now revealed in meagre part,
Yet drives all doubt away:
I stand in Christ, with sins forgiven;
And Christ in me, the hope of heaven!
My highest calling and my deepest joy,
To make His will my home.

There is a hope that lifts my weary head,
A consolation strong against despair,
That when the world had plunged me in its deepest pit,
I find the Saviour there!
Through present sufferings future's fear,
He whispers 'courage' in my ear.
For I am safe in everlasting arms,
And they will lead me home.

There is a hope that stands the test of time,
That lifts my eyes beyond the beckoning grave,
To see the matchless beauty of a day divine
When I behold his face!
When sufferings cease and sorrows die,
And every longing satisfied.
Then joy unspeakable will flood my soul,
For I am truly home.

Tuesday 20th OCTOBER, 2009
TO TEACH IS TO TOUCH A LIFE FOREVER

Dear everyone,

Today is my 63rd Birthday and right glad I am to see it. I have had a terrific day, believe me! As I reflect on the Lord's goodness to me across my life and its extension over these last months, I bow my head in worship and thanksgiving. How very privileged I am! I have wondered how to close this little book of letters and thought I would do so by first quoting from a letter I received amidst an avalanche of wonderful messages received this year. This very humbling letter was from Mark Russell, the current Chief Executive of the Church Army, who was awarded the British Gas Tomorrow's People Award for his cross community work, bringing Catholic and Protestant young people together across Northern Ireland. Again I say thank you to all who have so kindly prayed for my family and me and shown us the one thing that even outlasts faith and hope, namely love. The kindness shown to me by the Macmillan Cancer Support in counseling and practical help has also been priceless.

Whatever time is left to me, may God give me grace to use it to exalt Christ, and to glory alone - as Paul so movingly put it - in Christ's Cross.

My dear Derick,

I have just heard the news that you are battling with Leukaemia, and I wanted to write to assure you of my love and prayers. I was so saddened to hear this news, and I wanted to encourage you.

I am not sure if you remember me, but I used to come to the Crescent when I was at Queen's, from 1992-1995, and then worked as Youth pastor of the Methodist Church in Lurgan. You kindly asked me one praise evening at the Crescent to share my story with the congregation. We used to correspond as well and I still have all the lovely letters you sent me.

You have been a tremendous influence on my life, and taught me to teach the Bible with passion, humour and energy. I just wanted to let you know where I am now which I hope is a blessing to you. I am now 34 and am the CEO of the Church Army, a mission agency in the Anglican Church. I am a member of the Archbishop's College of Evangelists, and serve on the Governing Council of the Church of England. I travel across these islands and over the world as a conference speaker and preacher. God has given me a really significant ministry …

I pray for God's blessing for you, and his healing.
With my love,
Mark.

The second message I want to quote was from a little girl called Grace Wilson. Back in September this year I had the privilege of publicly thanking the congregation at Portstewart Baptist Church for their great kindness to me throughout my illness. They set out a massive card for people to sign for me on Easter morning this year. I wept in my isolation ward when I received it. It was wonderful not to be forgotten. When I sat down in the congregation that morning in September, Grace was sitting with her father, the artist and sculptor Ross, and she quickly wrote the following note and passed it to me before I spoke: it says it all!

Dear Derick,

It is good to see you at Church this morning. It is nice to be out and about. I pray for you every night.

Love,
Grace
Aged 8

Saturday 24th OCTOBER, 2009
AND FINALLY ...

Something to Rest On

Give me something to rest on,
When life's trials move in,
When heartaches encircle,
And the ice is thin,
When all hope seems darkened,
And the old landmarks fade,
Give me something to rest on,
An eternal aide.

Christ is my resting place,
My song in the night,
My guide through the breaking storm,
My unfading light,
The way to the Father's heart,
The truth without spin,
The life to sustain me,
When all else caves in.

Moses let Egypt's treasures go,
For greater riches by far,
Ruth's faith shone as a gleaner,
Long before Bethlehem's star,
The Lord was David's shepherd,
Despite the wolf's ploys,
Faith saw beyond present grief
To incomparable joys.

Away with all unbelief!
Begone doubt and fear!
No evil can ever snatch me,
With the Lord so near,
On through the valley,
To the mountaintop in sight,
Beyond lies the city,
Where the Lamb is the light !

On, on through deep sorrow,
Where tears blind my eyes,
On, on to a place prepared,
Beyond those dark skies,
The cross is my glory,
The Lord is my song,
His face I shall touch,
Before very long.

At those feet sorely wounded,
I will soon gladly fall,
Never once regretting,
Seeking to give him my all,
If I had a thousand lives,
He could have every one,
I am heading for the light,
That comes from behind the sun!

Derick Bingham

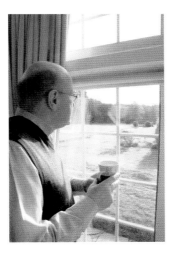

Derick's continuing letters can be read at

www.derickbingham.com